The Tomato Cookbook

2nd Edition

33 Amazing Tomato Dishes That You've Never Thought About!

by Olivia Rogers

Copyright © 2017 By Olivia Rogers
All rights reserved. No part of this book may be reproduced in any form without permission in writing from the author. No part of this publication may be reproduced or transmitted in any form or by any means, mechanic, electronic, photocopying, recording, by any storage or retrieval system, or transmitted by email without the permission in writing from the author and publisher.
For information regarding permissions write to author at Olivia@TheMenuAtHome.com
Reviewers may quote brief passages in review.

Please note that credit for the images used in this book go to the respective owners. You can view this at:
TheMenuAtHome.com/image-list

Olivia Rogers
TheMenuAtHome.com

Table of Contents

Introduction _____ 5
1. Tomato Butter Dip _____ 6
2. Stuffed Tomatoes _____ 8
3. Tomato Gravy _____ 10
4. Tomato & Corn Salad _____ 12
5. Tomato Bites _____ 14
6. Tomato Focaccia _____ 17
7. Watermelon Tomato Salad _____ 20
8. Tomato Egg Cups _____ 22
9. Tomato Gelato _____ 24
10. Tomato Sliders _____ 26
11. Tomato Pudding _____ 28
12. Tomato Consommé _____ 30
13. Tomato Snacks _____ 33
14. Tomato Blossoms _____ 35
15. Pomegranate Tomato Salad _____ 37
16. Grilled Tomato Toasts _____ 39
17. Oil Poached Tomatoes _____ 41
18. Grilled (Tomato Prosciutto) Cheese _____ 43
19. Tomato Vinaigrette _____ 45
20. Hot Tomatoes _____ 47
21. Salsa _____ 49
22. Crunchy Tomatoes _____ 51
23. Blue Cheese Tomato Salad _____ 53

24. Chunky Tomato Basil Sauce	55
25. Tomato Bread	57
26. Tomato Cucumber Feta Salad	59
27. Tomato Matzo Balls	61
28. Tomato Marmalade	63
29. Bacon Tomato Clams	65
30. Tomato Tarte Tatin	67
31. Polenta Gnocchi with Tomato Sauce	69
32. Tomato Watermelon Soup	71
33. Tomato Terrine	73
Final Words	76
Disclaimer	78

Introduction

When the tomato first made its way over to Europe from the New World, people were convinced the vibrant red color meant it was poisonous. For centuries, the tomato was simply considered a decorative plant. No one dared try eating it.

Once they finally became brave enough to taste it, there was no going back. Tomato quickly became a staple of many cuisines throughout Europe. Its popularity continues to this day, but most people greatly underestimate just how versatile this fruit is.

In this book, you'll learn how to prepare tomatoes in 33 different ways. From a traditional marinara sauce through to a refreshing tomato gelato! Now you can explore the full potential of this ingredient.

1. Tomato Butter Dip

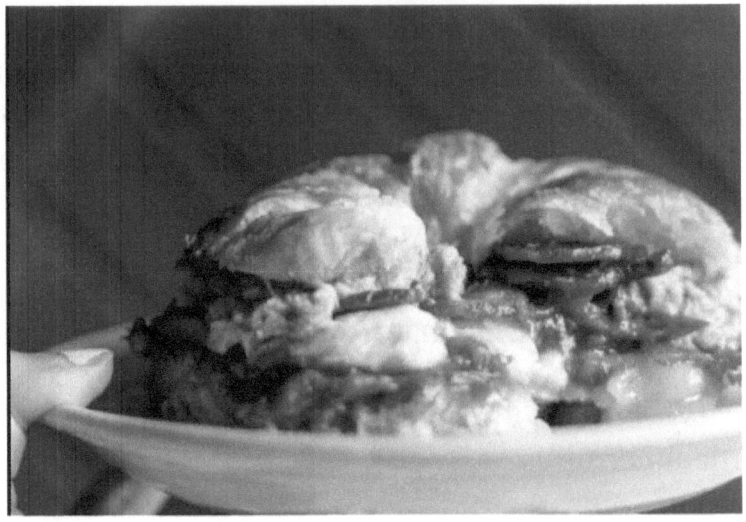

This is a great dip for veggies, chips, or chicken wings.

Ingredients

- Cherry Tomatoes
- Butter (softened)
- Salt

Method

1. Broil tomatoes until skins blister. Let cool. Pulse together with salt in a food processor.

2. Stir mixture into butter until well blended.

Tomato Trivia

The tomato is a tricky plant. Scientifically, it is a fruit. But according to the law, it is a vegetable. The tomato is the state vegetable of New Jersey and the state fruit of Ohio. But Arkansas beats both: the tomato is their state fruit and state vegetable.

2. Stuffed Tomatoes

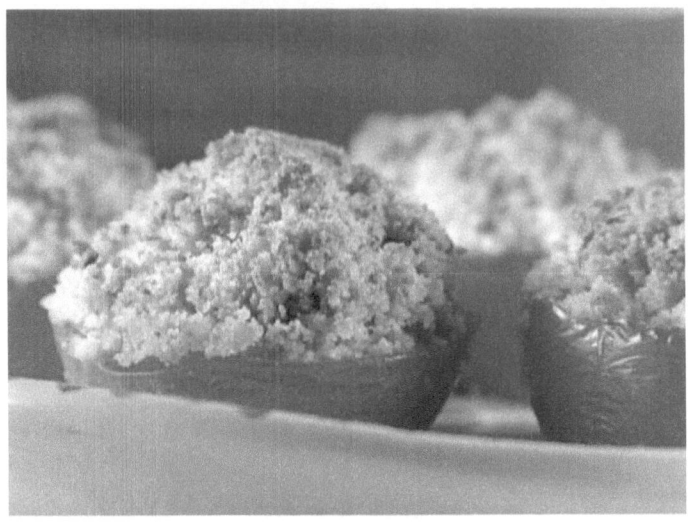

Transform tomatoes into edible bowls with this main course worthy dish.

Ingredients

- 1 loaf Italian Bread (crust removed)
- 2 cloves Garlic (chopped)
- 2 Tbsps. Capers
- 2 tsp Salt
- 6 Tbsps. Olive Oil
- 4 large Tomatoes

Method

1. Preheat oven to 250°F. Bake bread for 5 minutes on each side. Set aside. Raise temperature to 350°F. Cut bread into chunks and place in food processor. Pulse until crumbly but not pulverized. Set aside 1 cup of crumbs. Store the rest for later.

2. In a bowl, mix garlic, capers, breadcrumbs, salt, and olive oil. Halve the tomatoes and remove seeds. Fill the halves with breadcrumb mixture. Place on baking sheet. Bake for 20 minutes or until brown crust forms.

Tomato Trivia

Tomatoes are native to the Andes Mountains in Peru. The Aztec of Mexico believed that the seeds gave people the ability to see the future. When it was first brought to Italy, it was thought to be poisonous. The Spanish, on the other hand, thought it was an eggplant.

3. Tomato Gravy

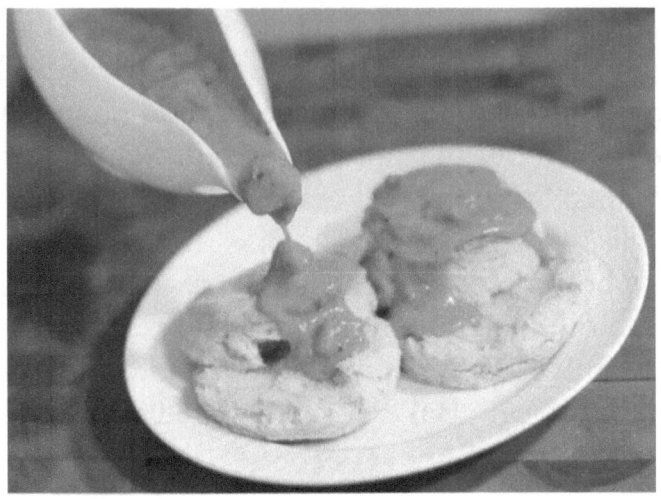

This healthier twist on gravy doesn't sacrifice flavor.

Ingredients

- ½ cup Butter
- 2 medium Onions (chopped)
- 2 tsp Thyme
- 2 Tbsps. Flour
- 1 (28 oz.) can Crushed Tomatoes
- 1/3 cup Scallions (sliced)
- 3 Tbsps. Heavy Cream

- 1 tsp Cayenne Pepper

- Salt & Pepper to taste

Method

1. Melt butter in a large pan on medium heat. Add thyme and onion. Cook 10 minutes, stirring often.

2. Add flour. Cook 3 minutes, stirring constantly. Add tomatoes with juice. Cook 30 minutes. Stir in cream, cayenne, scallions, salt, and pepper.

Tomato Trivia

Despite being native to South America, China has now become the largest producer of tomatoes today.

Tomatoes aren't just red. They can also be orange, yellow, green, pink, purple, brown, white, or black.

Today, there are more than 7,500 species of tomato.

4. Tomato & Corn Salad

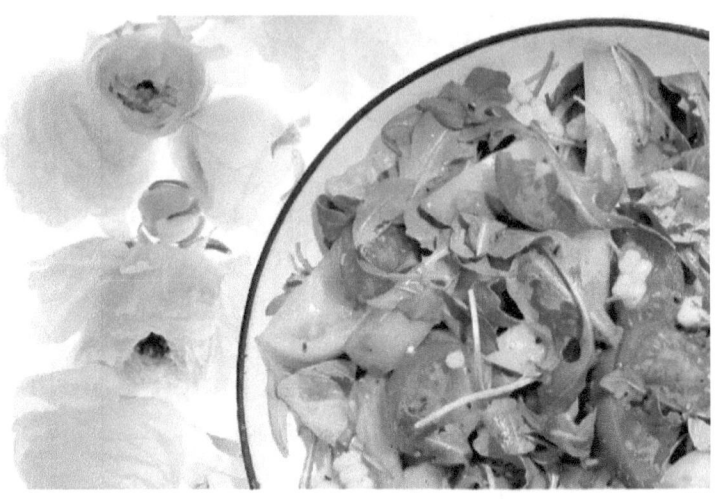

This simple salad proves that delicious doesn't have to be difficult.

Ingredients

- 6 large Tomatoes (diced)
- 20 ears Corn
- Salt, Pepper, Oil, Paprika to taste

Method

1. Prepare a grill on high heat. Blanch corn until bright yellow. Let air dry. Grill corn until slightly scorched on all sides.

2. Remove kernels from the cobs. Add the kernels, tomatoes, salt, pepper, and paprika to a large bowl. Stir. Add olive oil and mix until evenly coated.

Tomato Trivia

In Spain, there is an annual tomato fight. Over 40,000 people gather to pelt each other with tomatoes.

The Guinness World Record for the biggest tomato weighed in at a whopping 7 lbs. and 12 oz. (the size of a healthy newborn baby).

A single tomato plant at the Epcot Science project in Disney World produced over 32,000 tomatoes in a single year.

5. Tomato Bites

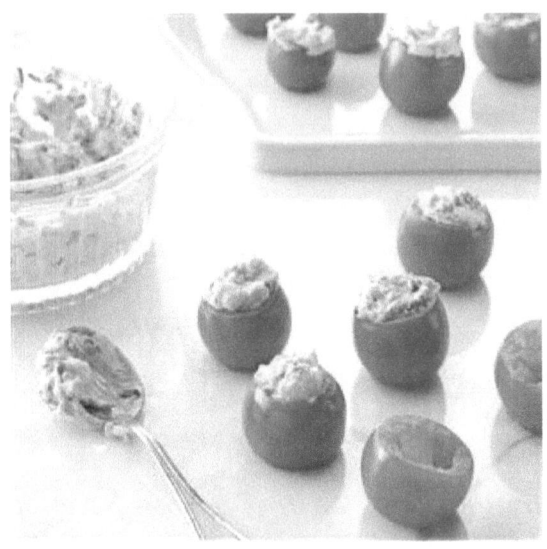

These simple yet flavorful snacks are the perfect treat for a summer day.

Ingredients

- 2 lbs. Tomatoes (sliced)
- 1 Scallion (sliced)
- 3 Tbsps. Olive Oil
- 2 Tbsps. Malt Vinegar
- ¾ tsp Brown Sugar
- Salt & Pepper to taste

Method

1. Whisk together salt, pepper, brown sugar, vinegar, and oil in a bowl. Arrange 1/3 of the tomatoes on a platter.

2. Drizzle a little of the oil mixture over them. Sprinkle some scallions on top. Repeat process twice to make 2 more layers.

Tomato Trivia

Eating a serving of tomatoes every day can reduce men's risk of prostate cancer by up to 43%.

Lycopene (the nutrient responsible for the cancer fighting effects) is best absorbed in fat so make sure you drizzle on a little extra olive oil!

Early research results suggest that tomatoes may even help combat the spread of cancer in patients who are already ill.

Read This FIRST - 100% FREE BONUS

FOR A LIMITED TIME ONLY – Get Olivia's best-selling book *"The #1 Cookbook: Over 170+ of the Most Popular Recipes Across 7 Different Cuisines!"* absolutely FREE!

Readers have absolutely loved this book because of the wide variety of recipes. It is highly recommended you check these recipes out and see what you can add to your home menu!

Once again, as a big thank-you for downloading this book, I'd like to offer it to you *100% FREE for a LIMITED TIME ONLY!*

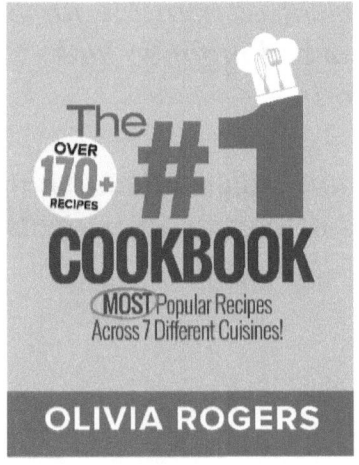

Get your free copy at:

TheMenuAtHome.com/Bonus

6. Tomato Focaccia

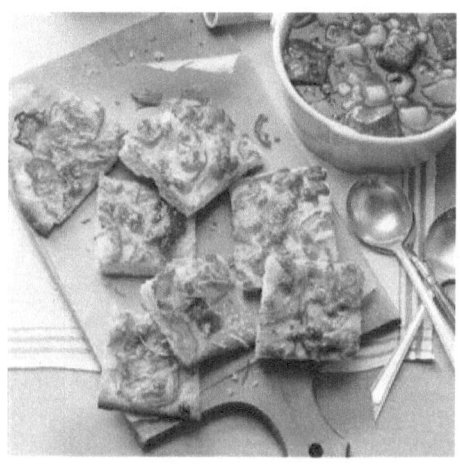

This wonderful focaccia is just the right blend of satisfyingly hearty and refreshingly light.

Ingredients

- ½ lbs. Potatoes (peeled, quartered)
- ½ lbs. Tomatoes (sliced)
- ½ cup Olive Oil
- 4 ¼ cups Flour
- 1 cup Warm Water
- 3 tsp Active Dry Yeast
- 1 Tbsp. Salt

- ½ tsp Sugar

- ¼ tsp Oregano

Method

1. Simmer potatoes in salt water for 10 to 15 minutes. Drain, cool, and mash. In a large bowl, mix sugar and warm water. Sprinkle in yeast. Let rest 5 minutes. Add mashed potatoes and ¼ cup oil. Mix until combined. Add flour 1 cup at a time and mix until a soft, sticky dough forms.

2. Knead on a floured surface 8-10 minutes. Place an oiled bowl and cover with oiled plastic wrap. Let rest in a warm place until doubled in size. Punch dough down and transfer to a greased baking dish.

3. Stretch dough so that it covers the bottom (may not fit exactly). Preheat oven to 425°F. Arrange tomatoes on top. Sprinkle with oregano, salt and ¼ cup oil. Bake until firm and pale golden (20 to 25 minutes).

Tomato Trivia

For women, the lycopene in tomato can help prevent cancer in the cervix, breasts and uterus.

If you're a smoker, eat a couple extra servings of tomato per day. Lycopene also helps guard against lung cancer.

Lycopene and vitamin A (both found in tomatoes) help make the skin more resistant to sun damage so make sure to eat extra in the summer.

7. Watermelon Tomato Salad

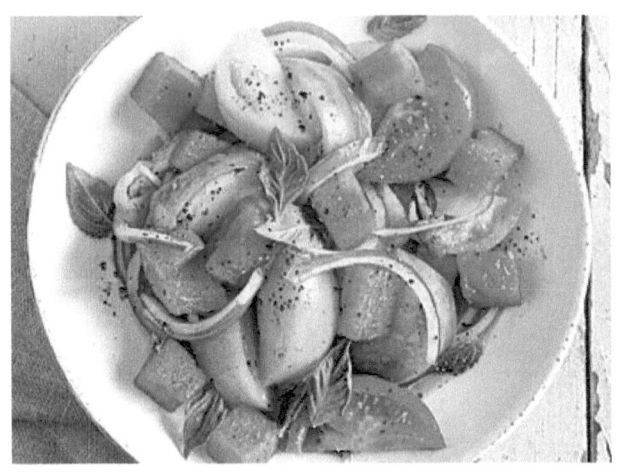

Leave your guests stunned with this mouthwateringly unique salad.

Ingredients

- 4 medium Tomatoes
- 1 small Cucumber
- 1 cup Watermelon (cubed)
- 1 Hass Avocado (diced)
- 3 Tbsps. Olive Oil
- 3 Tbsps. Balsamic Vinegar
- ¼ tsp Ground Coriander Seeds

- 1 Tbsp. Mixed Herbs (your preference)
- Salt & Pepper to Taste

Method

1. In a large bowl, combine watermelon, tomato, avocado, cucumber, herbs, and coriander. Mix well.

2. In a small bowl, whisk together vinegar, salt, pepper, and oil. Pour vinegar mixture over tomato mixture. Toss to coat.

Tomato Trivia

Americans eat an average of 24 lbs. of tomatoes each year. Over half of that amount is in the form of ketchup. That amount has increased by 30% over the past 20 years.

8. Tomato Egg Cups

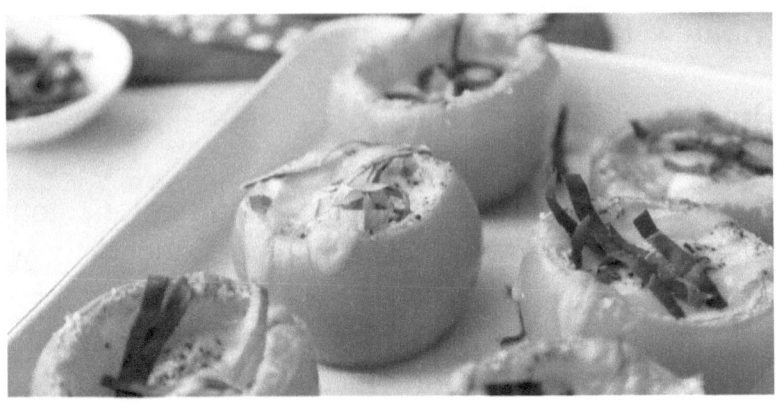

This ingenious dish makes a perfect breakfast.

Ingredients

- 4 medium Tomatoes
- 4 large Eggs
- 4 Tbsps. Cheddar Cheese (shredded)
- 4 slices Toast (cut in strips)
- Salt & Pepper to taste

Method

1. Preheat oven to 425°F. Slice the top 1/3 of each tomato. Set aside. Remove seeds. Place tomatoes in baking dish. Season with salt and pepper.

2. Crack an egg into each tomato. Put tomato tops back in place. Bake 10 minutes. Remove tops, sprinkle in cheese. Bake until bubbly (5-7 minutes). Serve with toast strips for dipping.

Tomato Trivia

*In German, the word for tomato (*Paridiesapfel*) translates to "apple of paradise." The scientific name (*solanum lycopersicum*) translates as "wolf peach." The word "tomato" comes from the original Aztec word* xitomatl *which literally translates as "plump thing with a navel."*

9. Tomato Gelato

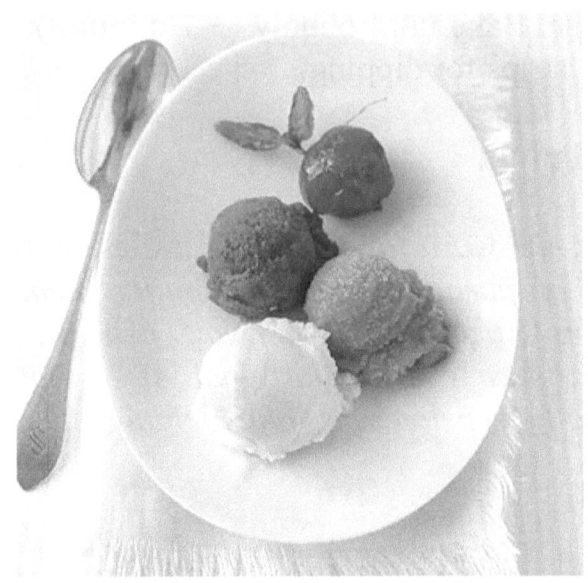

Pair this exquisite gelato with candied tomatoes and watch everyone come asking for the recipe.

Ingredients

- 2 lbs. Tomatoes (very ripe, chopped)
- 1 cup Simple Syrup (chilled)
- 1 pinch Salt

Method

1. Puree tomatoes until smooth. Strain through a fine sieve until you have 2 cups of puree.

2. Add simple syrup and a pinch of salt. Blend well. Transfer mixture to an ice cream maker. Process according to instructions.

Tomato Trivia

The acidity in tomatoes make them a perfect deep pore cleanser. Mash one up with some olive oil and give yourself a 20-minute facial. Mix a tablespoon of tomato juice with 2 drops of lime juice for a quick 10-minute pore-refining mask. Using either of these masks on a weekly basis will also help manage oily skin.

10. Tomato Sliders

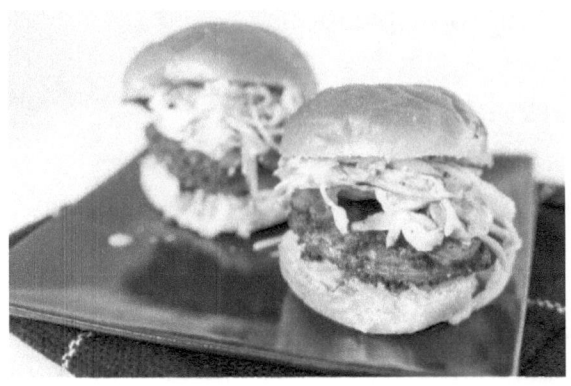

This recipe provides you with 3 different tomato-based appetizers so you're sure to please every palate.

Ingredients

- 8 large Tomatoes (in ½" slices)

- ¾ cup Hummus

- ¾ cup Black Olive Spread

- ¾ cup Pesto

- 2 cups Ricotta

- 3-4 Tbsps. Olive Oil

- Crusty bread

- Pepper to taste

Method

1. Spread hummus over 8 slices. Spread black olive spread over 8 slices.

2. Spread pesto over 8 slices. Arrange slices on a platter. Serve with bread slices and a bowl of ricotta with pepper and olive oil drizzled on top.

Tomato Trivia

A blend of tomato, aloe vera, and yogurt are the perfect homemade remedy for sunburns.

Tomato juice also happens to make an excellent shampoo and conditioner. Massage it into your scalp for 5 minutes to break apart buildup and rehydrate your scalp and hair.

Use a mask of tomato and honey on your face for 15 minutes to restore that natural youthful glow.

11. Tomato Pudding

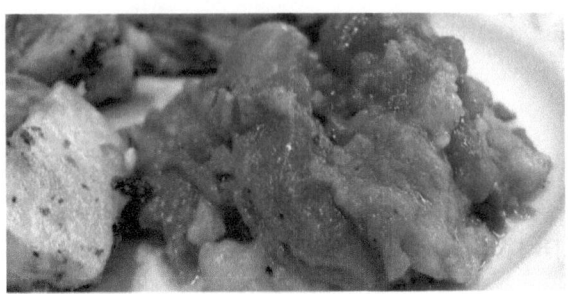

Put a new twist on tired old pudding with this savory tomato recipe.

Ingredients

- 4 ½ lbs. Tomatoes
- 1 (1 ¼ lbs.) Pullman Loaf (crust removed)
- 3 cloves Garlic (minced)
- 2 Tbsps. Olive Oil
- 2 ½ tsp Sherry Vinegar

Method

1. Blanch tomatoes for 1 minute. Remove skin. Blend garlic and salt to a paste. Halve tomatoes and remove seeds. Press seeds through a fine sieve to collect the juices. Discard seeds. Chop tomatoes and puree with collected tomato juice.

2. Heat 2 tablespoons olive oil in a large pan on medium-high heat. Add garlic past. Cook 1 minute. Remove from heat. Add a few spoonful's puree. When no longer bubbling, add remaining puree, salt, and pepper. Return to heat. Simmer 5 minutes, stirring occasionally.

3. Cool for 1 hour. Add vinegar. Cut bread into 12 triangle pieces and 3 circular pieces. Ladle ¾ cup tomato puree into soufflé dish. Place circular bread piece at the bottom. Fan 4 triangle pieces around until puree is covered completely. Repeat layers until filled (about 3 more times).

4. Cover top layer of bread with remaining puree. Cover with plastic wrap then place a plate just small enough to fit inside the dish on top. Weight down the pudding with 2 heavy cans or a 2 lbs. object. Chill 12 hours.

Tomato Trivia

Tomatoes continue to gain weight even after being harvested. Save a few cents at the store by getting unripe tomatoes and letting them ripen (and grow) at home!

In Victorian England, it was not socially acceptable to eat a tomato in public.

Tomato seedlings have been successfully grown in space.

12. Tomato Consommé

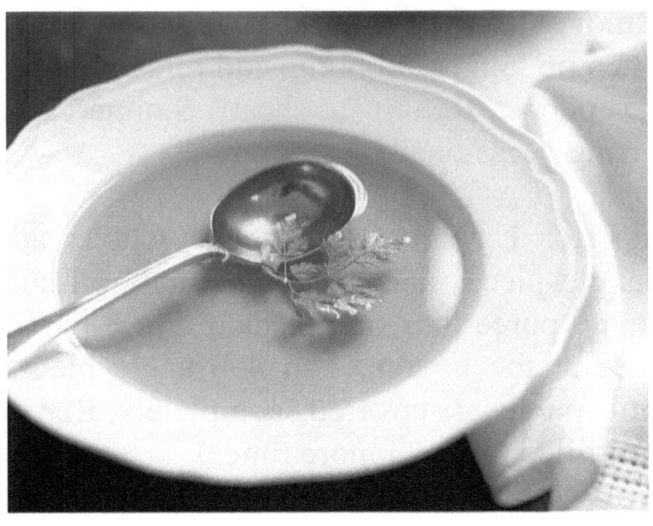

This consommé is light, refreshing, and simple to make.

Ingredients

- 5 lbs. Tomatoes (pureed)
- 10 oz. Pear Tomatoes (halved)
- 2 Onions (chopped)
- 1 ½ lbs. Fennel (halved lengthwise, cored, chopped)
- ¼ cup Parsley
- 8 large Egg Whites (chilled)
- 2 cloves Garlic (chopped)

- 2 Tbsps. Olive Oil

- 2 Tbsps. Basil

- 1 Tbsp. Tarragon

- ½ cup Crushed Ice

- 1 ½ tsp Sherry Vinegar

Method

1. In a large pot cook garlic, fennel, and onions in oil for 10-12 minutes. Stir in pureed tomato, salt, and pepper. Simmer 20 minutes. Pour mixture through a fine sieve into a large pan. Bring to a boil.

2. In a bowl, whisk together egg whites, ice, herbs, salt, and pepper until frothy. Pour egg white mixture into boiling broth, whisking constantly. Egg mixture will rise and form a "raft". Wait for the "raft" to bubble. Enlarge the holes made by bubbles to the size of a ladle.

3. Reduce heat and simmer 15-20 minutes (without stirring). Remove from heat. Ladle out consommé without disturbing the "raft". Place consommé in a fine sieve lined with damp paper towels set in a large glass bowl. Chill 1-2 hours. Before serving, toss per tomatoes with vinegar and salt. Serve on top of consommé.

Tomato Trivia

The leaves of the tomato plant are toxic.

The largest tomato vine is over 65 feet long. It can be found in England.

The largest tomato tree can be found in Disney World, but it was first discovered in Beijing.

13. Tomato Snacks

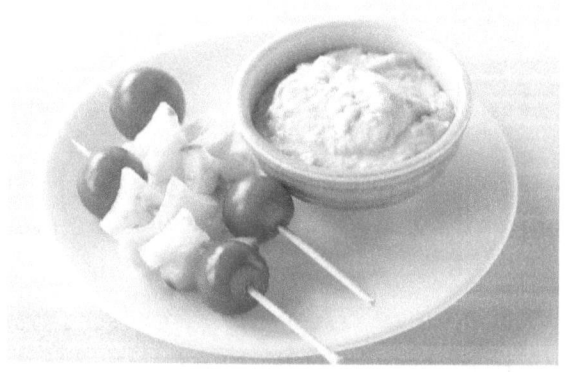

In just 10 minutes, you'll have a scrumptious snack that's ideal for summer picnics.

Ingredients

- 1 (8") Sourdough Round (cut into 3/4" slices)
- 4 small Tomatoes (halved)
- 2 cloves Garlic (halved)
- 4 Tbsps. Olive Oil
- Salt to taste

Method

1. Prepare grill for medium heat. Grill bread 1-2 minutes per side. Vigorously rub 1 side of each slice with garlic.

2. Do the same with tomato (until most of the pulp is absorbed in the bread. Brush bread with oil and sprinkle with salt.

Tomato Trivia

Storing tomatoes in the fridge makes them less nutritious and less flavorful. Keep them on the counter! The high vitamin C content in tomatoes is almost completely destroyed when cooked. However, the lycopene content is easier to digest in cooked tomatoes. So, eat a balance of raw and cooked tomatoes to get both.

14. Tomato Blossoms

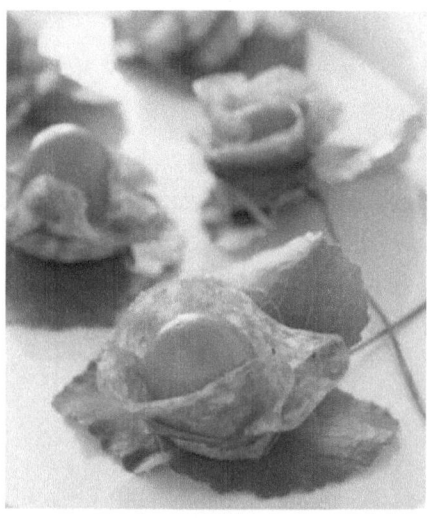

These adorable treats are easy to make and sure to put a smile on anyone's face.

Ingredients

- 18 Grape Tomatoes
- 18 Thin Slices Genoa Salami
- 18 long Fresh Chives
- 1/3 cup Peppered Boursin Cheese

Method

1. Stir basil and cheese until combined. Put ½ teaspoon of cheese mixture in the center of each salami round.

2. Press 1 tomato into the center of each cheese pile until stabilized. Gather salami up around the tomato and tie it in place with chive.

Tomato Trivia

Tomatoes are high in potassium making them a great pre-workout (or post-hangover) snack. They're also a good source of Vitamins A, K, and B vitamins (not to mention many minerals) so if you're looking for a well-rounded nutritious snack—the tomato is the answer. Lycopene also prevents wrinkles!

15. Pomegranate Tomato Salad

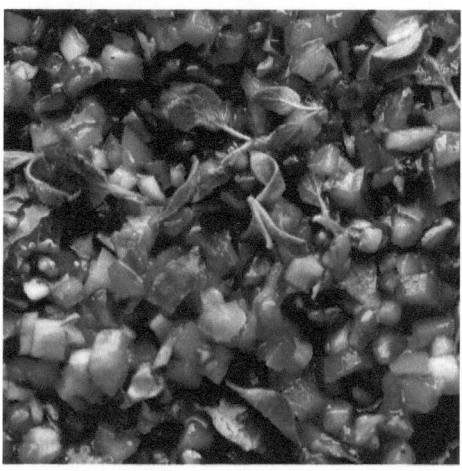

Impress your guests with this salad that's not just boldly flavored but a visually stunning masterpiece.

Ingredients

- 2 2/3 cups Cherry Tomatoes (red and yellow, diced)
- 1 1/3 cup Plum Tomatoes (diced)
- 1 lbs. medium Tomatoes (diced)
- 1 Red Pepper (diced)
- 1 Red Onion (diced)
- 1 cup Pomegranate Seeds
- 2 cloves Garlic (crushed)

- 1 ½ Tbsps. Molasses
- ¼ cup Olive Oil
- 2 tsp White Wine Vinegar
- 1 Tbsp. Oregano
- ½ tsp Allspice
- ½ tsp Salt

Method

1. In a large bowl, combine tomatoes, onion, and red pepper. In a small bowl, whisk together vinegar, molasses, garlic, olive oil, allspice, and salt.

2. Pour this over tomato mixture and mix until evenly coated. Arrange mixture with juices on a platter. Sprinkle pomegranate seeds and oregano over the top.

Tomato Trivia

The calcium and vitamin K in tomatoes help fight osteoporosis. The chromium helps stabilize blood sugar levels. The Vitamin A prevents age related macular degeneration in the eyes.

16. Grilled Tomato Toasts

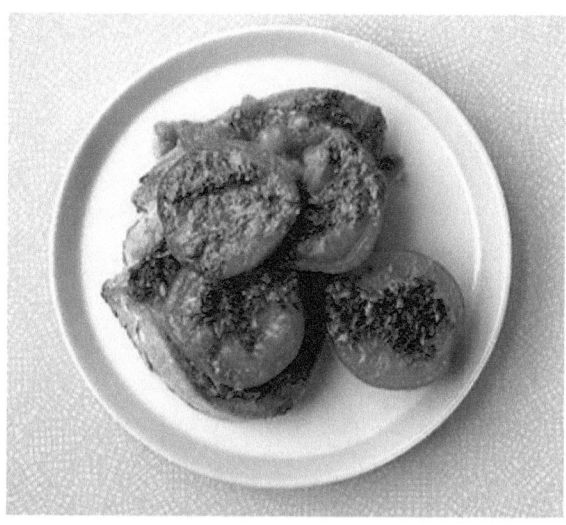

These no-hassle treats are the perfect appetizer or light lunch.

Ingredients

- ¾ lbs. Small Tomatoes
- 8 slices Crusty Bread
- 10 oz. Ricotta
- 1 cup Mixed Fresh Herbs (your preference)
- 1 clove Garlic (chopped)
- 6 Tbsps. Olive Oil

- 1 Tbsp. Red Wine Vinegar

- Salt & Pepper to taste

Method

1. Combine garlic and salt into a paste. Transfer to a bowl. Whisk in 2 tablespoons oil and the vinegar. Add tomatoes, salt, and pepper. Toss to coat. Prepare grill to medium-high heat.

2. Brush both sides of bread with olive oil. Grill 1-2 minutes per side. Add herbs to tomato mixture. Toss until evenly mixed. Spread ricotta on top of toast. Top with tomato mixture.

Tomato Trivia

Getting your daily dose of tomatoes will reduce your risk for kidney stones and gallstones. Tomatoes have anti-inflammatory effects making them a great pain reliever. Tomatoes are low in calories but highly satisfying making them an excellent addition to your weight loss program.

17. Oil Poached Tomatoes

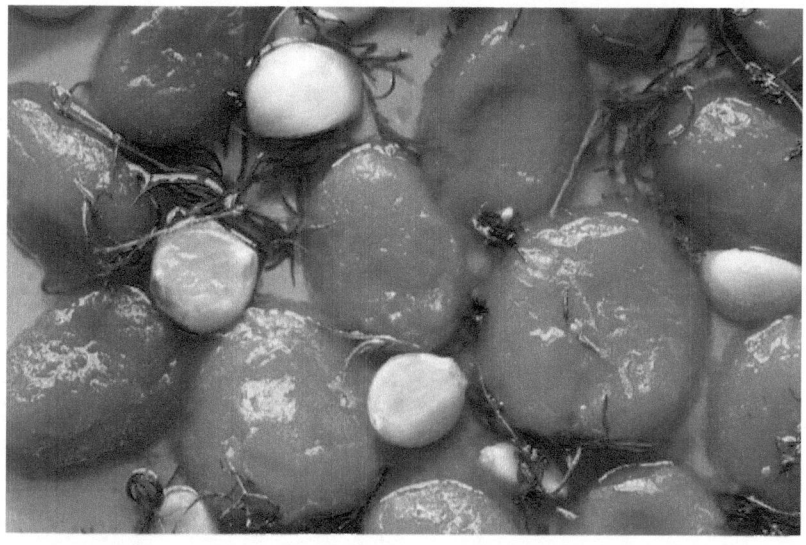

Tomatoes are the unchallenged star of this wonderfully elegant dish.

Ingredients

- 1 lbs. Plum Tomatoes (halved)
- 1 head Garlic (cloves separated)
- 1 cup Olive Oil
- 2 sprigs Rosemary
- 2 sprigs Thyme
- Salt to taste

Method

1. Preheat oven to 300°F. Toss together rosemary, garlic, oil, thyme, and salt in a baking dish.

2. Bake tomatoes until soft (35-45 minutes). Remove skins. Discard herbs.

Tomato Trivia

Tomatoes should be a big part of your diet if you're diabetic as they help your body process glucose better. The choline in tomatoes helps your body break down and absorb fat. It also helps you sleep better.

18. Grilled (Tomato Prosciutto) Cheese

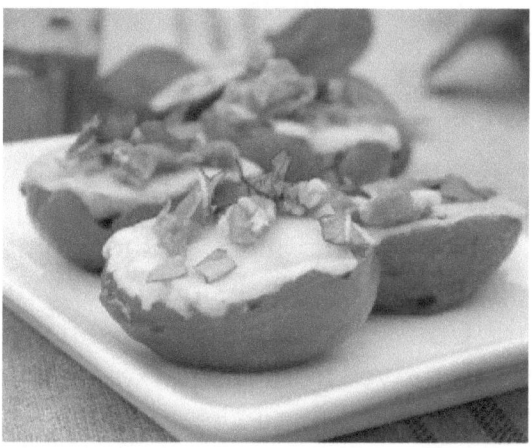

Turn that regular grilled cheese into a restaurant quality lunch with these simple modifications.

Ingredients

- 8 slices Whole Grain Bread
- 8 slices Prosciutto
- 2 cups Cheddar (shredded)
- ½ can Tomatoes
- 1/8 cup Red Onion (chopped)
- 4 Tbsps. Olive Oil
- 1 Tbsp. Red Wine Vinegar

- 1 clove Garlic (minced)
- ½ tsp Honey

Method

1. Preheat oven to 350°F. In a small pot on medium heat, cook onion, garlic, and tomato until it resembles a jam (about 15 minutes). Add honey and vinegar. Cook 15 minutes. Season with salt and pepper. Remove from heat. Arrange half of your bread slices on a baking sheet.

2. Top each slice with ¼ cup cheese and 1 slice prosciutto. Bake 3 minutes. Spread tomato jam on top of the prosciutto. Top with remaining bread slices. Heat 1 tablespoon oil in a pan. Cook each sandwich for 3 minutes per side.

Tomato Trivia

The high potassium in tomatoes also helps to lower blood pressure. Fiber, potassium, and vitamin C work together to protect your heart from disease and heart attack. Tomatoes help maintain collagen in the skin and prevents damage from not only the sun but also pollution, smoke, and the aging process.

19. Tomato Vinaigrette

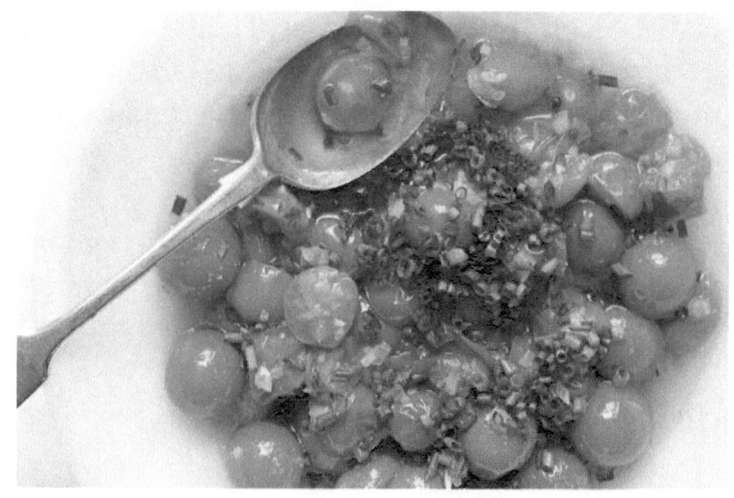

Liven up any salad with this delicious and simple vinaigrette.

Ingredients

- 1 lbs. Cherry Tomatoes
- 3 Tbsps. Olive Oil
- 1 Tbsp. Red Wine Vinegar
- 2 Tbsps. Chives (chopped)
- 1 Shallot (chopped)
- Salt & Pepper to taste

Method

1. Halve ½ lbs. cherry tomatoes. Heat 1 tablespoon oil in a pan on medium heat. Add shallot. Cook 4 minutes, stirring often. Add all the tomatoes (halved and whole). Cook 4-6 minutes.

2. Mash some of the tomatoes with a spoon. Add vinegar and 2 tablespoons oil. Season with salt and pepper.

Tomato Trivia

Tomatoes are a great source of folic acid (especially important for pregnant women). Folic acid may also treat depression. The lycopene is even more effective than it is in other sources because, in the tomato, it's teamed up with its 3 carotenoid cousins (alpha, beta, and lutein).

20. Hot Tomatoes

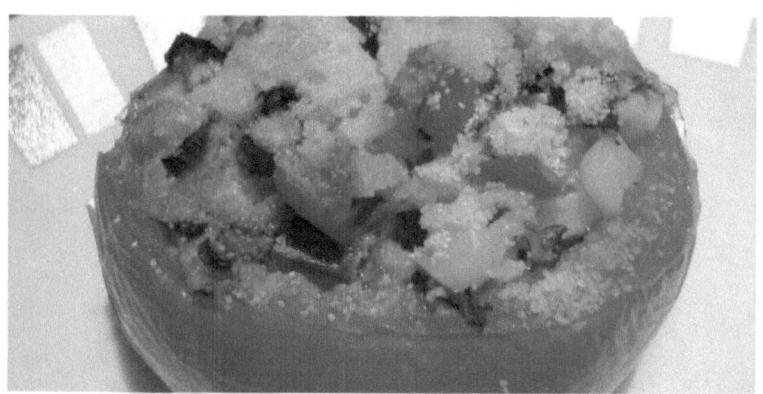

These simple yet bold appetizers are sure to make an impression at any party.

Ingredients

- Cherry Tomatoes
- Horseradish
- Mayonnaise
- Fresh Herbs (your preference)

Method

1. Core the cherry tomatoes and scoop out centers. In a bowl, combine mayonnaise and horseradish to taste. Spoon mixture into tomatoes. Top with fresh herbs.

Tomato Trivia

Combining tomatoes with fats (like mayonnaise, olive oil, or avocado) increases your absorption of the tomato's nutrients by 15%.

Breastfeeding women should eat lots of tomato sauce to help their newborn get plenty of lycopene.

The majority of the nutrients are housed in the tomato's skin so avoid peeling them.

21. Salsa

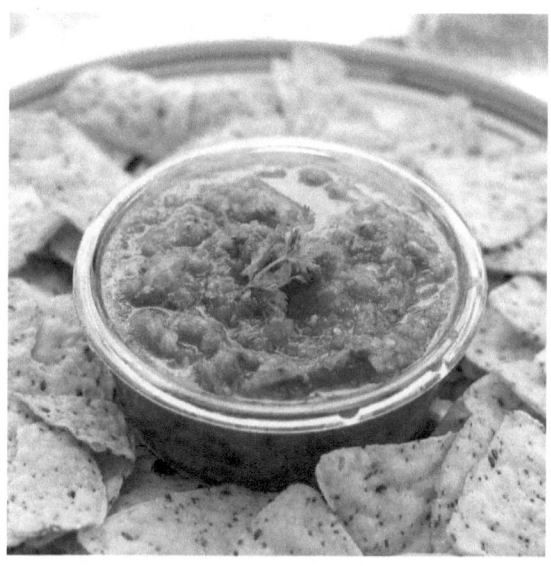

This isn't just any old salsa. Avocado and serrano chili provide unexpected and bold flavors.

Ingredients

- Tomatoes (diced)//
- Corn Kernels
- Avocado (diced)
- Serrano Chili (minced)
- Cilantro (chopped)
- Salt to taste

Method

1. Combine all ingredients in a bowl. Mix well.

Tomato Trivia

Coumaric acid and chlorogenic acid (found in tomatoes) protect your body from carcinogens (like pollution and smoke) so city dwellers and smokers alike should be eating tomatoes on the d daily. The vitamin A in tomatoes keeps your hair strong and glossy. It's also great for your teeth.

22. Crunchy Tomatoes

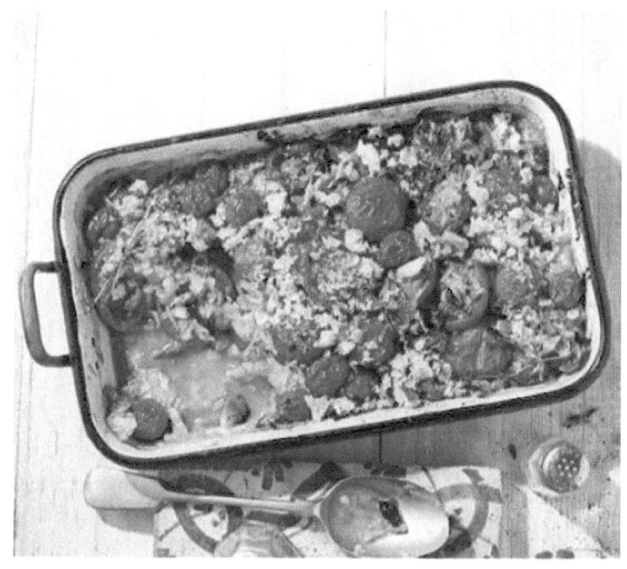

Replace your chips and popcorn with these delicious snacks.

Ingredients

- Tomatoes (sliced)
- Seasoned Breadcrumbs
- Olive Oil

Method

1. Arrange tomato slices in a pie dish. Pour in olive oil until partially submerged. Let soak 30 minutes. Turn slices over after 15 minutes.

2. Remove from oil (save oil for salad dressing). Press one side of each slice into breadcrumbs.

Tomato Trivia

Tomatoes that have green rings of unripe flesh around the stem are sweeter and more flavorful than the kind that are uniformly colored.

Plum tomatoes are the most used for ketchups and sauces.

Of the 7,500 species of tomato, only 13 of them are wild.

23. Blue Cheese Tomato Salad

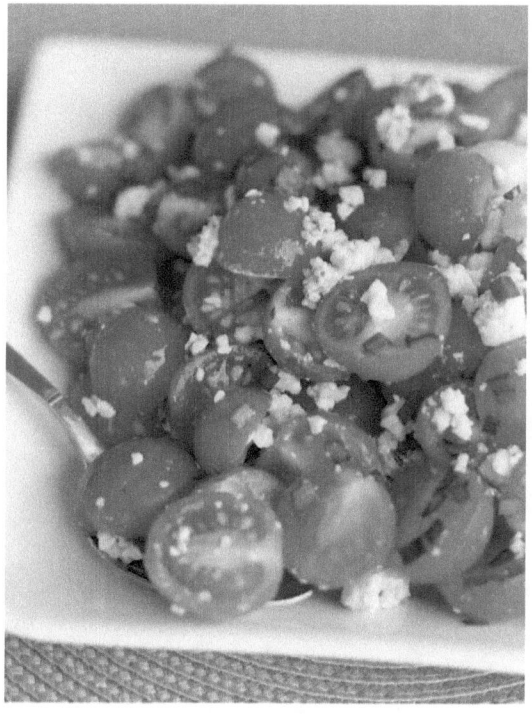

This salad is the perfect quick fix to any meal that's missing a side dish.

Ingredients

- Tomatoes (cut in wedges)
- Chives (chopped)
- Blue Cheese Dressing
- Pepper to taste

Method

1. Arrange tomato wedges on a platter. Drizzle blue cheese dressing over. Sprinkle chives and pepper on top.

Tomato Trivia

To disprove the myth that tomatoes were poisonous, local New Jersey resident Robert Johnson ate an entire basket of them on the courthouse steps in 1820.

After a childhood prank, Ronald Reagan didn't eat a single tomato for the next 70 years.

Tomatoes are the key ingredient in 78% of America's most popular recipes.

24. Chunky Tomato Basil Sauce

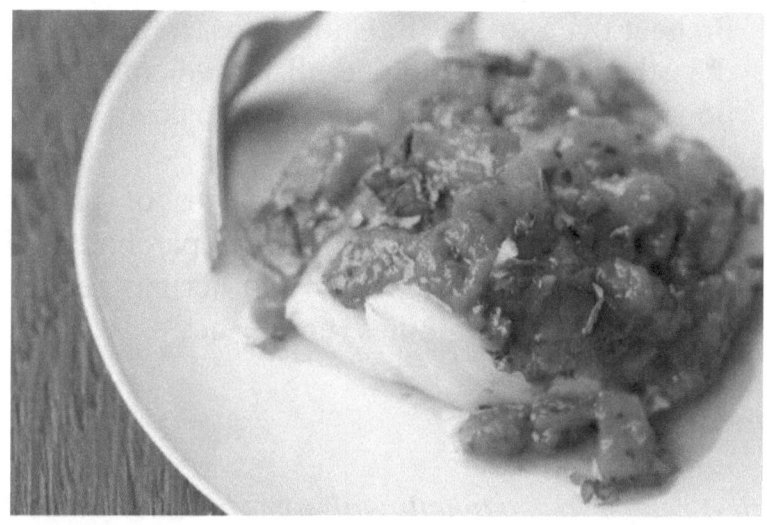

Use this sauce recipe to top pasta, fish, rice, polenta, or as a base for other sauces.

Ingredients

- 2 lbs. Cherry Tomatoes
- 7 cloves Garlic (sliced)
- 8 sprigs Basil
- 5 Tbsps. Olive Oil
- 1 Shallot (chopped)
- Salt & Pepper to taste

Method

1. Preheat oven to 350°F. Chop 1 lbs. tomatoes. Halve the other pound. Combine all ingredients in a large bowl with 4 tablespoons oil. Toss to coat.

2. Line a baking sheet with 3 pieces of parchment paper. Spoon mixture on top of parchment. Fold paper over the mixture and crimp edges to seal. Bake 25-30 minutes (until saucy).

Tomato Trivia

The first recipe for spaghetti with tomato sauce dates back to 1790 by an Italian chef working in Russia.

You can gauge nutrition value by color. The deeper the red, the more lycopene it contains.

The smallest tomatoes are tomberries (less than 1" in diameter).

25. Tomato Bread

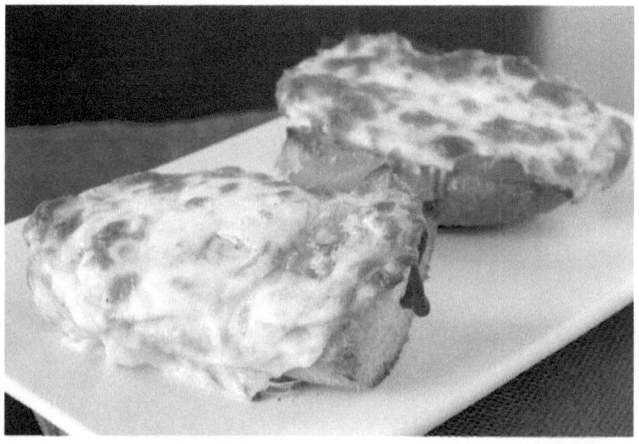

Say goodbye to plain old white bread and try out this rich, bold tomato bread with a touch of basil.

Ingredients

- 2 ½ cups Whole Grain Flour
- ¾ cup Warm Water
- 1 package Active Dry Yeast
- 3 Tbsps. Tomato Paste
- 2 Tbsps. Basil (dried)
- ¼ cup Parmesan Cheese (grated)
- 1 Tbsp. Sugar

- 1 Tbsp. Olive Oil

- 1 tsp Salt

- 1 tsp Crushed Red Pepper Flakes

Method

1. In a large bowl, dissolve yeast in warm water. Stir in basil, parmesan, sugar, salt, pepper flakes, tomato paste, oil, and 2 cups flour. Mix until combined. Add the rest of the flour 1 tablespoon at a time until a stiff dough is formed. Knead on floured surface 3-5 minutes. Place in an oiled bowl. Cover with oiled plastic wrap.

2. Let rise in a warm place until doubled in size. Punch dough down. Knead 1 minute. Shape into a loaf. Place on greased baking sheet. Cover and let rise until doubled in size. Preheat oven to 375°F. Cut an X on the top of the loaf. Bake 40 minutes (or until golden).

Tomato Trivia

While safe for humans, too many tomatoes can be toxic for dogs. They can be toxic to you as well, if eaten unripe (or if you eat the leaves and stems). But a puree of ripe tomatoes can help treat urinary tract infections.

26. Tomato Cucumber Feta Salad

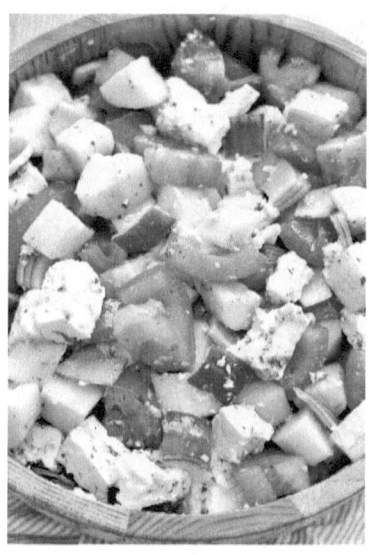

Add a refreshing and colorful side dish to your meal with this exquisitely simple salad.

Ingredients

- 2 lbs. Cucumber (chopped)
- 1 lbs. Tomatoes (chopped)
- 1 (7oz.) package Feta Cheese (crumbled)
- 1 bunch Scallions (chopped)
- 1 cup Olives (pitted, halved)
- ½ cup Fresh Mint (chopped)

- 6 Tbsps. Olive Oil

- ¼ cup Fresh Lemon Juice

- Salt & Pepper to taste

Method

1. Combine veggies and half of the feta in a large bowl. Mix in mint. In a small bowl, whisk together oil and lemon juice. Add salt and pepper. Pour dressing over salad. Toss to coat. Sprinkle remaining feta crumbles on top.

Tomato Trivia

The modern word for the fruit is almost identical in every language because they use a variation of the original Aztec "xitomatl."

There are 4 species that stand out with the highest lycopene content: New Girl, Jet Star, Fantastic, and First Lady.

There's no reason to spring for organic. Studies show that the species is more important than the method grown when it comes to nutrition.

27. Tomato Matzo Balls

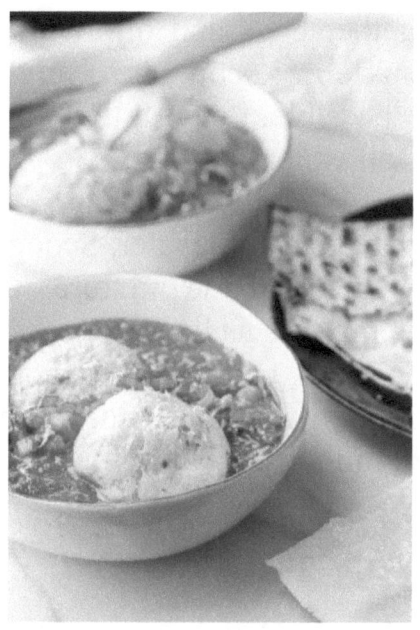

These rich matzo balls are perfect in a simple broth or covered in a creamy sauce.

Ingredients

- 2 large Eggs
- 1 large Egg White
- 3 Tbsps. Tomato Paste
- ¾ cup Matzo Ball Mix
- 2 Tbsps. Olive Oil

Method

1. Whisk together eggs and oil. Whisk in the tomato paste. Sprinkle in ½ cup matzo mix. Stir but mix as little as possible. Let chill in the fridge 20 minutes. Boil water.

2. Wet your hands in cold water. Scoop out a small ball (ping pong size) of the mixture with your hands. Disturb the mixture as little as possible. Gently form the lump into a ball. Reduce boiling water to a simmer. Drop balls into the simmering water. Simmer 20 minutes.

Tomato Trivia

Tomatoes help prevent both constipation and diarrhea. Tomatoes contain phytonutrients that prevent blood clotting and lower bad cholesterol. New studies are showing that lycopene also prevents bone tissue from degrading.

28. Tomato Marmalade

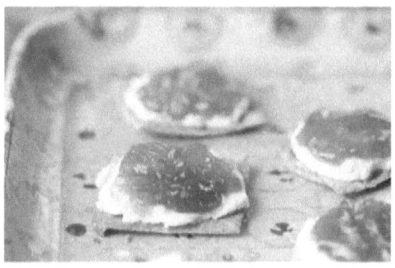

Spread this on toast, crackers, or pancakes for a sweet topping with a surprising note of tomato.

Ingredients

- 3 ½ lbs. Sweet Tomatoes
- 1 lbs. Lemons (seeded, sliced)
- 1 lbs. Oranges (seeded, sliced)
- 4 lbs. Sugar
- 4 oz. Fresh Lemon Juice
- 1 large pinch Saffron
- 1 Cinnamon Stick

Method

1. Place lemon and orange slices in a stainless-steel pot. Submerge in cold water. Place pot on high heat.

Cover. Bring to a boil. Let boil 1 minute. Drain. Return slices to pot. Cover in 1" cold water. Bring to a boil over high heat. Reduce heat and simmer 35 minutes.

2. Bring a pot of water to a boil. Drop the tomatoes in. Cook 1-2 minutes until skins loosen. Drain. Remove tomatoes skins. Use hands to tear tomatoes into chunks. Place citrus and tomato in a glass or plastic container and refrigerate overnight. Pour mixture into a large preserving pan. Add cinnamon stick. Stir well.

3. Bring to a boil over high heat. Cook 30 minutes or until it sets. Do not stir until it foams. Then, stir every few minutes. Marmalade is done when it looks glossy and contains tiny bubbles throughout. Remove a small spoonful with a frozen spoon to check for a jelly consistency. Remove cinnamon stick. Pour marmalade into sterilized mason jars. Seal the jars.

Tomato Trivia

Eat cooked tomatoes before bed. Lycopene improves sleep quality. Tomatoes are one of the few foods that can be used as both a fruit and a vegetable. In addition to versatility in the kitchen, tomatoes are also the base of many home remedies.

29. Bacon Tomato Clams

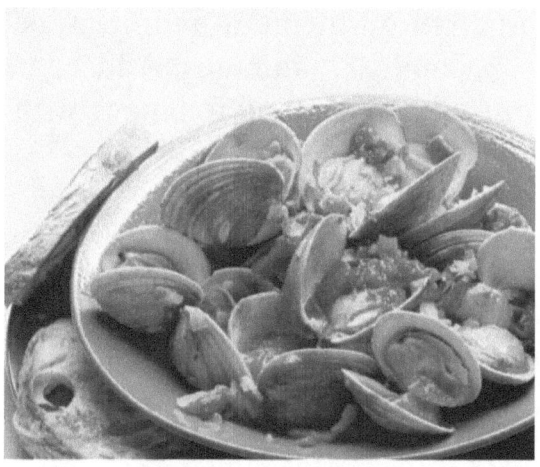

This unique dish creates a complex body of delicious flavors.

Ingredients

- 6 slices Bacon
- 1 (28oz.) can Diced Tomatoes
- 6 lbs. Clams
- ¼ cup Parsley
- 3 cloves Garlic
- 1 Onion (chopped)
- ½ cup Roasted Red Bell Peppers (from jar, drained)

Method

1. In a large pot on medium-high heat, add bacon and onions. Cook 8 minutes. Add garlic. Stir 1 minute. Add peppers and tomatoes with juice. Bring to a boil. Stir to combine.

2. Add clams. Cover and boil 8-10 minutes, stirring occasionally. Stir in parsley. Serve.

Tomato Trivia

A virgin Bloody Mary is an effective remedy for morning sickness.

Gargling with tomato juice twice daily can treat mouth ulcers.

Those with eczema or sun sensitivity should include tomato in every meal.

30. Tomato Tarte Tatin

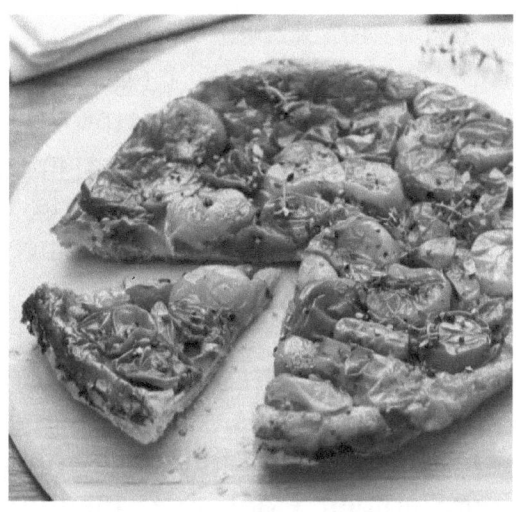

Finally treat tomato like the fruit it is with this exquisitely intriguing dessert.

Ingredients

- 1 ¾ lbs. Plum Tomatoes
- 1 sheet Puff Pastry
- ¾ cup Sugar
- 3 Tbsps. Butter (softened)
- 1 tsp Vanilla Extract
- Whipped Cream

Method

1. Preheat oven to 425°F. Boil water in a large pan. Drop in tomatoes. Cook 1 minute. Peel tomatoes. Core, halve, and remove seeds. Spread butter over bottom of large pan. Sprinkle in sugar. Arrange tomatoes in single layer on top of butter. Place pan over medium heat. Cook 25 minutes, stirring occasionally.

2. Remove from heat. Drizzle vanilla over tomatoes. Top with pastry rounds. Tuck in edges of pastry with knife. Cut 2-3 slits into each round. Bake until pastries are golden. Cook over medium heat for 10 minutes. Remove from pan onto platter.

Tomato Trivia

Place a slice of tomato on minor burns or wounds to soothe and heal them.

1-2 fresh tomatoes on an empty stomach can help reduce redness in the eyes.

An ointment of tomato paste, lemon juice, and turmeric can be used as an effective treatment for dark circles.

31. Polenta Gnocchi with Tomato Sauce

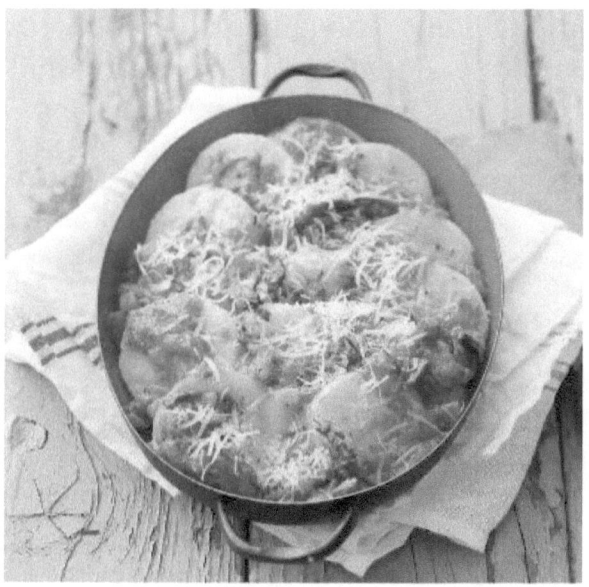

Polenta puts an interesting twist on this Gnocchi topped with a variation on the chunky sauce described earlier in this book.

Ingredients

- Prepared Polenta
- Chunky Tomato Basil Sauce (see above)
- ½ cup Mushrooms (sliced)
- ¼ cup Parmesan (grated)
- Pepper to taste

Method

1. Prepare chunky tomato basil sauce according to recipe. Line a baking sheet with aluminum foil. Grease with olive oil. Spread prepared polenta across in a smooth layer. Refrigerate 2-4 hours. Stamp out small polenta rounds.

2. Preheat oven to 400°F. Roll polenta into gnocchi shape. Grease a baking dish with olive oil. Arrange polenta rounds in dish so that they are slightly overlapping. Spoon in sauce generously. Bake 30 minutes. Remove from oven. Sprinkle with parmesan, parsley, and pepper.

Tomato Trivia

Eat a blend of 6 oz. tomato paste with 3 cloves minced garlic as a remedy for diarrhea or infections (viral or bacterial).

Drink tomato juice regularly if you're anemic.

A facial mask made of tomato paste done weekly will minimize acne scars and reduce the number of breakouts.

32. Tomato Watermelon Soup

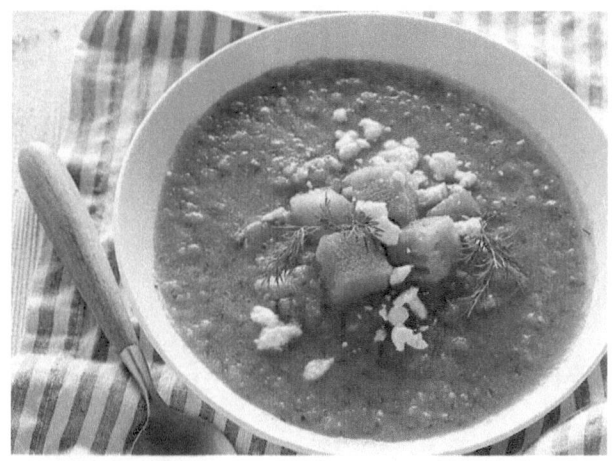

Tomato and watermelon combine to create a bold yet refreshing flavor in this soup.

Ingredients

- 2 cups Watermelon (seeded, cubed)
- ½ lbs. Tomatoes (quartered)
- 2 Tbsps. Unsalted Almonds (ground)
- 1 Tbsp. Black Olives (pitted, chopped)
- 2 Tbsps. Feta (crumbled)
- 1 Tbsp. Fresh Lemon Juice
- 1 Tbsp. Red Wine Vinegar

- ½ Shallot (quartered)

- 2 tsp Fresh Mint

- 1 tsp Olive Oil

Method

1. Pulse together all the ingredients (except feta, olives, and mint) in a food processor until smooth. Top with crumbled feta, olives, and mint.

Tomato Trivia

Planting basil next to your tomatoes will increase your tomato yield by about 20%. Planting onions or garlic near your tomatoes will help ward off pests. Tomatoes and Carrots are the best pals in the garden. They each strengthen the other.

33. Tomato Terrine

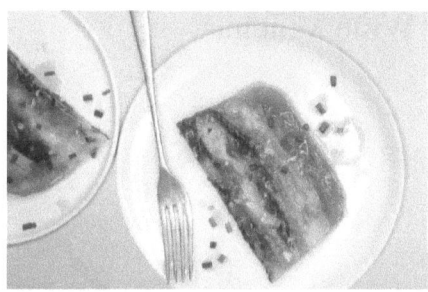

This summery dish is a perfect starter or light lunch on a hot afternoon.

Ingredients

- 6 lbs. Tomatoes (varying colors, peeled, quartered)
- 2 Carrots (chopped)
- 1 leek (sliced)
- 1 stalk Celery (chopped)
- 1 Shallot (halved)
- 1 clove Garlic
- 10 sprigs Parsley
- 10 Peppercorns
- 1 ½ Tbsps. Plain Gelatin

- ¼ cup Chives (sliced)

- 2 tsp Red Wine Vinegar

- 1 tsp Salt

- Olive Oil

Method

1. In a large pan, boil 3 cups of water with carrots, leeks, celery, shallots, garlic, parsley, peppercorns, and oil. Reduce heat to medium. Simmer 15 minutes. Strain through a fine sieve. Preserve liquid. Discard solids. Fillet the tomato wedges. Reserve the seeds and juice.

2. Press seeds and juice through fine sieve to collect ½ cup juice. Sprinkle the gelatin into the juice. Let stand 10 minutes. Add stock liquid from earlier. Whisk vigorously until gelatin dissolves. Stir in vinegar, salt, and chives. Pour into a greased baking dish that's lined with plastic wrap.

3. Pour ½ cup liquid into pan. Chill 40 minutes. Arrange 1 layer filleted tomato wedges on top of chilled liquid. Drizzle 2 tablespoons of liquid over them. Repeat these layers until ingredients are used up. Cover with plastic wrap. Weigh down the top with another pan with 2-3 heavy cans on top. Chill 6 hours.

Tomato Trivia

*The scientific name (*solanum lycopersicum*) meaning "wolf peach" comes from old werewolf myths in which this family of plants was used to transform into a werewolf.*

Throwing rotten tomatoes was a popular alternative to booing a bad performance in the 19th century.

Indigo Rose, Sun Black and other purple or black tomatoes contain anthocyanin which is a powerful antioxidant.

Final Words

I would like to thank you for downloading my book and I hope I have been able to help you and educate you about something new.

If you have enjoyed this book and would like to share your positive thoughts, could you please take 30 seconds of your time to go back and give me a review on my Amazon book page!

I greatly appreciate seeing these reviews because it helps me share my hard work!

Again, thank you and I wish you all the best with your cooking journey!

Last Chance to Get YOUR Bonus!

FOR A LIMITED TIME ONLY – Get Olivia's best-selling book *"The #1 Cookbook: Over 170+ of the Most Popular Recipes Across 7 Different Cuisines!"* absolutely FREE!

Readers have absolutely loved this book because of the wide variety of recipes. It is highly recommended you check these recipes out and see what you can add to your home menu!

Once again, as a big thank-you for downloading this book, I'd like to offer it to you *100% FREE for a LIMITED TIME ONLY!*

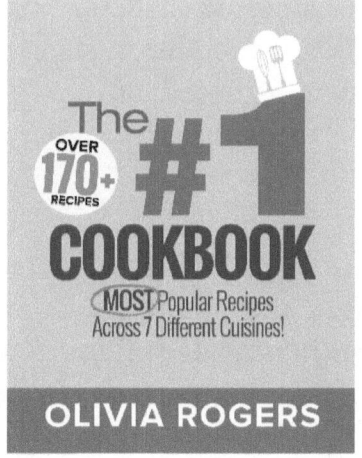

Get your free copy at:

TheMenuAtHome.com/Bonus

Disclaimer

This book and related site provides recipe and food advice in an informative and educational manner only, with information that is general in nature and that is not specific to you, the reader. The contents of this book and related site are intended to assist you and other readers in your personal efforts. Consult your physician or nutritionist regarding the applicability of any information provided in our information to you.

Nothing in this book should be construed as personal advice or diagnosis, and must not be used in this manner. The information provided about conditions is general in nature. This information does not cover all possible uses, actions, precautions, side-effects, or interactions of medicines, or medical procedures. The information in this site should not be considered as complete and does not cover all diseases, ailments, physical conditions, or their treatment.

No Warranties: The authors and publishers don't guarantee or warrant the quality, accuracy, completeness, timeliness, appropriateness or suitability of the information in this book, or of any product or services referenced by this site.

The information in this site is provided on an "as is" basis and the authors and publishers make no representations or warranties of any kind with respect to this information. This site may contain inaccuracies, typographical errors, or other errors.

Liability Disclaimer: The publishers, authors, and other parties involved in the creation, production, provision of information, or delivery of this site specifically disclaim any responsibility, and shall not be held liable for any damages, claims, injuries, losses, liabilities, costs, or obligations including any direct, indirect, special, incidental, or consequences damages (collectively known as "Damages") whatsoever and howsoever caused, arising out of, or in connection with the use or misuse of the site and the information contained within it, whether such Damages arise in contract, tort, negligence, equity, statute law, or by way of other legal theory.

www.ingramcontent.com/pod-product-compliance
Lightning Source LLC
Chambersburg PA
CBHW021131080526
44587CB00012B/1228